# Child Autism and Music Therapy

A Research to give parents new perspectives and possibilities for intervention with a natural art therapy

# Table of contents:

# Chapter II – MUSICOTHERAPY

2.1 Definitions and principles of music therapy

2.2 Historical notes

2.3 The figure of the music therapist

2.4 Active and receptive music therapy: the intervention techniques used

2.5 Principles of music therapy

   2.5.1 The principle of ISO

   2.5.2 The intermediary object

   2.5.3 The integrating object

   2.6 Areas of intervention


# Chapter III – MUSICOTHERAPY AND AUTISM

3.1 Music and communication

3.2 Music therapy applied to autism

3.3 Benenzon's model in infantile autism

3.4 Therapeutic dynamics

3.5 The intervention project

**CONCLUSIONS**

# INTRODUCTION

In the last twenty years on the national scene, as already for some time abroad, art therapies are emerging with increasing importance, or at least diffusion, and in particular music therapy which has now become a known and accredited practice.

If we talk about music therapy today, we usually refer to an area of rehabilitation or treatment, which presupposes that we are in the sphere of discomfort.

With my book, I wanted to carry out a research study on how music can become a valid therapeutic tool to help in the life, development and communication management of children suffering from the autistic syndrome.

It is extremely difficult to establish contact with these children, but the therapeutic use of music can be a more direct form of communication when the possibility of using traditional linguistic codes is lost. Music therapy, as a technique for opening communication channels, thus becomes the ideal therapy to approach autistic children.

Autism is a subject that has always fascinated and intrigued me; a closed and impenetrable universe that, after years of research, traditional and modern approaches are allowing us to understand and treat therapeutically. I tried to understand what is hidden in the mysterious and particular world of the autistic child; I wanted, therefore, to deepen this particular condition.

The image that struck me most during my study path was the metaphor of the extraterrestrial by Therese Joliffe *"If normal people were on another planet with alien creatures, they would probably feel scared, they wouldn't know what to do to adapt and they would surely have difficulty understanding what the aliens think, feel and want and to answer all this correctly. Autism is like that. If everything suddenly changes on this planet, a normal person would worry, especially if he didn't understand the meaning of this change. This is how the autistic feel when things change "*.

This metaphor highlights the diversity of the autistic person, which, however, cannot in any way affect the dignity and value of the person; indeed, it enhances their originality.

My thesis is divided into five parts: three chapters, the introduction, and conclusions.

In the first chapter, starting with Leo Kanner's definition of autism, I will present a general picture of the characteristics and typical aspects of the pathology. I will present a historical overview of the studies conducted on this type of disability, the various historical stages will be stated and, in particular, I will refer to a significant stage, namely, 1943, the year in which Leo Kanner (a hospital psychiatrist at the hospital of John Hopkins of Baltimore), carried out a study on eleven children: The picture he defined was that of infantile autism understood as a syndrome distinct from other psychiatric conditions.

Subsequently I will focus on epidemiology, on the etiopathogenetic mechanisms that include the interpretative models of the clinic, the neurobiological bases and the causal factors.

I will continue with the classification of diagnostic criteria by referring to the currently used nosography systems such as DSM-IV-TR and ICD-10.

Finally, I will focus on the possible presence of disorders associated with autism such as mental retardation and epilepsy.

In the "chapter II" of my work, I will introduce music therapy through the definition given by Rolando Benenzon, an Argentine neurologist and psychotherapist considered one of the pioneers of music therapy. I will go back over the origins of the discipline, the uses of music in ancient civilizations and the path that it has marked both in the spiritual field and in the health field up to the first forms of research in the scientific field to reach, finally, the official birth of music therapy as a scientific methodology.

I will introduce the figure of the music therapist and, subsequently, I will focus on the most significant relationships in music therapy, such as those between patient and music and patient-music therapist. I will continue to describe the intervention techniques used and the fundamental principles of music therapy; I will, therefore, quote the theoretical principles of the ISO on which the sound identity of each individual is based, the intermediary object and the integrating object.

I will conclude this chapter with an exposition of the main areas that make use of the music therapy intervention: the educational-preventive field, the habilitative-rehabilitative field, and the (psycho) therapeutic field.

The third and final chapter of my thesis aims to validate the therapeutic power of music capable of reducing the extent of the expression and communication disorder of the child with the autistic syndrome. Music therapy allows communication with a channel different from the usual and can improve behavior in the relationship with oneself and with others.

In this chapter, particular attention will be paid to the exposition of the music therapy model in infantile autism by Rolando Benenzon which develops around the research of ISO and the intermediary object and includes three levels of work: the regression level, the level of communication and the level of integration.

Subsequently I will address how the therapeutic dynamics develop in music therapy and, subsequently, the intervention project that makes use of two fundamental technical elements: the ideal laboratory of music therapy and the instruments. It will follow how music therapy sessions are structured.

I will conclude this chapter with an article taken from an Italian local gazette "The case of Giovanni: the first words after 15 years" where a mother's story attests to the progress made by her autistic son thanks to the help of music therapy.

# Chapter I AUTISM

## 1.1 Definition

*"It is an innate inability to form the usual emotional contact with people, biologically determined [...], just as other children come into the world with innate physical or intellectual handicaps."*

Autism is a complex neurodevelopmental disorder with onset in the first three years of life. Initially autism was considered to be of psychosocial origin, but the most current research and experiences have increasingly highlighted the neurobiological aspect.

It manifests itself with serious alterations in the areas of verbal and nonverbal communication, social interaction and imagination with narrow, repetitive and stereotyped patterns of behavior.

"Being autistic translates, with varying degrees of gravity, into the inability to communicate with the world of others, to establish a visual-attentive contact with others, to imitate their behavior and to understand their thoughts, emotions, and feelings".

## Background

Autism derives from the Greek autòs which means "itself" because, as a particular model of psychic structure, characterized by isolation: a child with autism seems to live in his world, showing little interest in others, and a lack of social awareness.

The term autism was used for the first time in the early twentieth century, in 1916, by Eugene Bleuler, the father of modern psychiatry, in the field of schizophrenia, about adult mental patients, to indicate a behavior represented by the closure in itself, avoidance of the other and isolation.

He modified the concept of schizophrenia by identifying an important symptom of withdrawal from structured social life in the self, as he observed in schizophrenic adults.

According to Bleuer, autism had to describe the narrowing of relationships with people and the outside world to the exclusion of one's self.

Thus began the idea of a particular symptomatic manifestation that accompanied the most serious psychological pathologies.

The first publications on autism as a specific disorder date back to the forties when two Austrian doctors Leo Kanner and Hans Asperger used, independently of one another, the term Autism.

Leo Kanner deserves the credit for having first published a work hypothesizing the existence of infantile autism as a syndrome distinct from other psychiatric conditions.

In 1943 Kanner, who worked in the United States and was director of the department of child psychiatry of John Hopkins hospital in Baltimore, published an article in the magazine entitled Nervous Child.

Autistic disorders of affective contact, where he describes eleven children aged between two and ten years, nine males and two females, who present a characteristic complex of symptoms, different from that observed in other forms of mental development deficit.

This article was the first attempt to explain autism from a theoretical point of view and is still today a reference point for research on this disorder.

The essential characteristics of the disorder introduced by Kanner and currently still considered valid are:

- autistic isolation;

- the desire for repetitiveness;

- the preserved islands of cognitive capacity;

he argued that social isolation constituted the main characteristic shared by the children he observed: "the most obvious fundamental disorder, pathognomonic, is the inability of children to relate to people and situations in the usual way [...]. Profound isolation dominates all behavior ". Within a general incapacity to communicate, serious problems of language and social relations are particularly present. "The sounds and movements of the child and all its performances are as monotonously repetitive as they are his verbal expressions. There is a clear limit to the variety of its spontaneous activities. The child's behavior is governed by an anxiously obsessive desire to preserve repetitiveness ". Kanner concluded by saying that these children came into the world with an innate inability to form the usual, biologically provided, emotional contact with people, just as other children come into the world with innate physical or intellectual handicaps.

The Austrian doctor Hans Asperger, a year after Kanner's first article was published, described a group of children who presented with a disorder that he called autistic psychopathy.

The social isolation, the stereotypy and the resistance to the changes of routine surprisingly followed the characteristics of the eleven children described by Kanner. Like Kanner, Asperger suggested that there was a disturbance of contact at some deep level of affects and / or instincts. Both highlighted the characteristics of communication, difficulties in social adaptation, stereotyped movements and excellent intellectual abilities in restricted areas. Asperger's subjects were distinguished by being characterized by a form of concrete thought, an obsession with certain subjects, excellent memory and often eccentric behavioral and relational modalities.

Children with Asperger's Syndrome can become high-functioning individuals with normal IQ or above normal.

However, Asperger identified three important areas in which his subjects differed from those of Kanner:

1. area of language: Asperger's subjects had a fluent speech. In Kanner's subjects, on the other hand, there was no language or it was not used in a communicative manner;

2. area of motor skills: in Kanner's opinion, children were only awkward concerning tasks of complex motor skills; according to Asperger they were both in complex and fine motor skills.

3. area of learning: Kanner thought that children showed higher performance when they learned in a mechanical, almost automatic way; Asperger instead described them as abstract thinkers.

In conclusion, two different diagnostic frameworks were configured: Kanner's classic Autism and Asperger's Syndrome. However, the similarities between the two diagnostic frameworks are so remarkable that, in 1994, Happè wondered if Asperger's syndrome was not "a label for all autistic people with relatively high IQs".

After the first paper, in 1955 Kanner shifted his attention to the behavioral characteristics of the parents of these children and, in particular, of the mother considered generally cold, detached, more attentive to the improvement of his career and social position than to the care of children. Moreover, he assumed a greater incidence of autism in higher socio-cultural classes.

The considerations on the hypothetical coldness and the social class of the parents are today considered outdated; the conception of autism, despite having undergone some adjustments over the years, still maintains the behavioral description defined by Kanner in 1943.

In the twenty years following Kanner's observations, thanks to the latter's theoretical approach, psychodynamic theories were the main point of reference in the study of autism.

The authors of the psychodynamic approach directed their efforts to investigate the possibility that the autistic syndrome was due to an alteration of the mother-child relationship.

Bettelheim was undoubtedly one of those who set up his work based primarily on this interpretation. The deficits of the person with autism, for Bettelheim, were therefore not organic but were triggered as a reaction to the parents' lack of affection and attention. These children retreated into a form of isolation that protected them from external influences. Bettelheim has greatly influenced the promotion of this theory by coining the term "refrigerator-mothers" to designate the coldness and detachment with which mothers of autistic children cared for their children.

In 1967, the year in which Bettelheim wrote "The empty fortress", the lack of research and scientific methods to understand autism, had contributed to the spread of numerous interpretations without scientific foundation.

These theories have been largely refuted by subsequent epidemiological studies, thanks to the advent of new, more refined study techniques of the anatomic-functional brain structure.

Starting in the 1960s, criticism of the psychodynamic model, accused of unfairly blaming parents, grew stronger. The parents of children with autism did not show pathological or personality traits significantly different from those of unaffected children.

Around the sixties, Rimland was the first to argue systematically that the cause of the autistic syndrome was not to be charged to the parents, but that the disorder had an organic basis. According to the author, in fact, autism was caused by morphological and organic-based functional alterations. The result was the organicist approach, which sought to identify organic alterations underlying the syndrome.

The position of psychiatrist Michael Rutter is significant, which in 1978 further specifies the picture described by Kanner, identifying some typical symptoms of infantile autism through a comparative study of autistic children and children with other types of disorders.

Rutter's attention focused on the following fundamental parameters:

- an onset within the first thirty months of age;

- an inability to develop social relationships, with avoidance modalities of a bodily, visual and auditory nature

- absence of language or presence of a particular form of language delay with the presence of echolalia and pronominal inversion;

- obsessive desire to keep the environment always in the same way with excessive worries and violent resistance to change;

- a tendency to various ritual and compulsive phenomena

Rutter also pointed out that about three-quarters of children with autism also have mental retardation.

Despite the variety of elements gathered congruent with this hypothesis, one, in particular, has not yet been isolated that can be considered as characteristic of all forms of autism, so much so that currently one is led to believe that there is no single autism, but that in this category are, instead, included various pathologies and symptomatic manifestations caused by different organic causes.

A year later, in 1979, Lorna Wing and Judy Gould carried out a study aimed at defining the distinctive features of autism.

The study showed that at the base of autism there was a combination of three impairments, with different degrees of severity, that Wing and Gould called triad of impairments:

- impairment of social interaction;

- impairment of social communication;

- Impairment of social imagination.

Autism was therefore identified as a syndrome characterized by a triad of disorders and no longer as an association of arbitrarily chosen symptoms.

The Camberwell study also examined the evaluation of social disorder from a qualitative point of view, distinguishing three different types of people with autism:

- the reserved ("halo") quite similar to the patients described by Kanner;

- the liabilities ("passive") above all towards the surrounding environment;

- the strange socially active ("active but odd"), but with incongruent and unusual behaviors.

Each of these types of behavior can be found in the same child in different situations and at different ages.

**Epidemiology**

The most recent and reliable studies, which use the standard criteria of diagnostic manuals, show an incidence of autism cases of about 60 per 10,000 subjects, with an estimate of cases in the classical form of 8-30 cases per 10,000.

Currently, at least one child in 1,000 shows some typical characteristics of autism even if it does not manifest the complete behavioral pattern of the symptomatic triad.

It has been widely established that the incidence rate is 4-5 times higher in males than in females with an average ratio of 4: 1. In Asperger's syndrome, this disparity seems more evident with a ratio of about 15: 1. The reason for this obvious difference has not yet been clarified, however, it has been observed that in low capacity levels the number of affected males is smaller, while the affected females show a more serious cognitive deterioration. The scarcity of females at high levels of capacity could indicate a biological origin of autism. Several hypotheses have been put forward; it could be a greater vulnerability of the male sex or, on the contrary, the presence of protective factors in the female sex. In females, probably, a more severe organic lesion and a greater genetic influence are needed. A more recent study has confirmed that sex differences are more correlated with IQ scores than the clinical severity of autism.

These findings are consistent with the results of other studies that have shown that autism per se is relatively independent of intellectual abilities and learned skills.

## Etiopathogenetic mechanisms

Autistic syndrome has long been considered a pathology of the so-called higher functions of the brain and initially classified among the psychoses.

The causes of autism are currently unknown. The nature of the disorder, in fact, involving complex mind-brain relationships, does not make possible the reference to the sequential etiopathogenetic model, commonly adopted in medical disciplines: etiology -> pathological anatomy -> pathogenesis -> symptomatology. It should also be considered that autism, as a syndrome defined exclusively in behavioral terms, is configured as the final common pathway of pathological situations of various kinds and with different etiologies.

The etiology, pathological anatomy, and pathogenesis are posed about autism, as three areas of research still indistinct, as the causal relationships between them are currently undefined.

The countless studies dedicated to the topic can be placed in three research areas:

- the interpretative models of the clinic (the pathogenesis);

- the neurobiological bases (pathological anatomy);
- causal factors (etiology).

**Interpretative models of the clinic**

The attempt to explain the alterations observed in the field of communication and social interaction in children with autism led, in the eighties, to various neuro-cognitive theories among which the most accredited are: socio-affective theory, the theory of the mind, the theory of weak central coherence and the theory of a deficit in executive functions.

The socio-affective theory starts from the assumption that the human being is born with an innate predisposition to interact with the other. For Hobson, autism is a disturbance of intersubjectivity and presupposes that at the basis of this disorder there is a lack of emotional relationship with the world, in association not only with deficiencies indirect social perception but also with difficulties in categorizing and relating to the world in relation to itself...

According to the socio-affective theory there would exist in autism an innate inability, biologically determined, to interact emotionally with the other. This incapacity, according to a cascade reaction, would lead to the inability to learn to recognize the mental states of others, the impairment of symbolization processes, the language deficit and the deficit of social cognition. Regarding specifically the linguistic anomalies in people with autism, Hobson has hypothesized that they are a direct consequence of the disturbances of socialization, of the absence of an affective and relational propensity towards people.

The term Theory of mind was introduced for the first time in 1979 by Woodruff and Premack to indicate the continuous activity of attribution to others of mental states such as beliefs, desires, deceptions, discoveries and so on, as well as the ability to understand, explain, to predict the behavior of others governed by such intentional states.

In the eighties Baron-Cohen, Leslie and Frith hypothesized that the deficit of social interaction in children with autism was due to an impairment of intersubjectivity, that is, of the ability to attribute to other intentions, desires, feelings, and beliefs; a deficit, therefore, in the theory of the mind.

The discovery of one's own mind and that of others would be a progressive evolutionary achievement.

In 1987 Leslie even considered that there could be a module of the theory of mind, which would be activated on a maturing basis and which would be substantially independent of experience. It would seem that in the normal child the theory of the mind begins to develop around the age of four.

This interpretation, however, is supported by logical and speculative arguments and not by substantial empirical-experimental evidence. Highlighting, however, a process of development of the theory of mind in the child, leads to the need to research its various evolutionary stages. In other words, those particular behaviors that can be considered precursors of the theory of the mind must be carefully analyzed. Among these, the earliest in development seems to be shared attention, intentional proto-declarative communication and the game of fiction. Children are thus able to attribute to others' thoughts, desires, and fantasies and this leads them to be able to foresee their behavior.

The ability to read emotions, desires, and beliefs, to organize them in a system of knowledge develops and refines the capacity of representation and meta-representation of children. In particular, this latter capacity, which represents the very essence of the theory of mind, allows the cognitive system to construct descriptions of hypothetical events.

The autistic child presents very substantial deficiencies in the processes of shared attention, of proto-referential communication, in the game of fiction and, consequently, fails to adequately develop a theory of the mind.

As for shared attention and proto-referential communication, they tend not to follow the adult's line of sight and not to look alternately at the adult and an interesting object. Moreover, both in observational and experimental conditions, these children show themselves capable of producing and understanding the gesture of indicating with a requested function, while they rarely use the same gesture with a declaratory function, ie trying to direct the adult's attention to it.

On the ability to implement symbolic games on the part of autistic children, there is a substantial agreement among the various researchers in considering these behavioral modalities severely compromised due to deficiencies in the formation of meta-representations.

The theory advocated by Baron-Cohen is that autism would be linked to an inability of the child to access a theory of mind, which is derived from the hypothesis of blindness of the mind in the autistic child. According to this approach, the autistic child would be incapable of understanding and reflecting on one's own and others' mental states and, consequently, of understanding and predicting the behavior of others.

Weak Central Coherence Theory proposes that autistic subjects have a preference for a detail-based information processing style.

According to Uta Frith, this cognitive style can also be present in non-autistic people, ie it constitutes a more global cognitive phenotype that confers advantages in the superior processing of perceptual details.

In the normal cognitive system there is the innate ability to integrate fragmented information into coherent or meaningful global representations for the context; this capacity seems reduced in autistic children and, consequently, their action processing systems are characterized by detachment.

Normally the operation of central coherence allows human beings to give priority to the understanding of meaning, so in a sentence we grasp the meaning of the message, which is even better remembered if it can be inserted in a wider context. This ability in the context of central processes, defined as a push towards central coherence, is a natural characteristic of the cognitive system and it is hypothesized that it is strongly lacking in people with autism. This deficit can explain, according to Frith and Happè, both the deficiencies that are found and the islands of abilities sometimes surprising. This type of functioning was proved by experiments in which the results showed high performance of autistic children in tasks that require the isolation of stimuli and favor detachment, compared to their poor performance in tasks that require the connection of stimuli and promote consistency.

Detachment or fragmentation into meaningless activities becomes inevitable consequences, given the limited capacity to achieve central coherence or meaning and this could also be the cause of the social deficit.

Finally, the executive functions are the functions that regulate the processes of planning, control, and coordination of the cognitive system and which govern the activation and modulation of the most elementary schemes and processes. In executive functions, three main components can be identified: the capacity for inhibition, the working memory and the ability to generate new strategies. The three executive components indicated above can be damaged relatively independently; in fact, the one most affected in autistics is the ability to generate new solutions.

The deficit of executive functions involves problems in the self-organization of any behavior that is not habitual and, therefore, could explain the presence of stereotyped behaviors and restricted interests. In fact, the behavior of autistic people often appears rigid and inflexible. However, these executive deficits are not specific to autism and the correlation with social disorders is still not clear. These deficits are probably related to impaired cortical mechanisms affecting the prefrontal cortex. Furthermore, the presence of similar cases within family groups could highlight a common genetic basis.

Sally Ozonoff argues that frontal injury can be considered an important but not sufficient condition for the development of autism; in fact, for the syndrome to manifest itself the presence of other cognitive deficits or neurological dysfunctions is necessary.

## Neurobiological bases

As far as the neurobiological causes underlying the disorder are concerned, the research areas are numerous and still in development. Studies on anatomical structures, and the neurotransmitters involved, have not reached univocal and definitive results.

The current neurobiological hypothesis defines autism as "a neurobiological disorder of predominantly localized polygenetic development in the central nervous system and associated with multi-organ involvement".

## Anatomical structures

In 1990 the morphological studies of the central nervous system conducted through computerized axial tomography were revealed, according to the judgment of Lelord and Sauvage, quite variable and often disappointing. In fact, some non-specific morphological alterations are reported, such as the uni or bilateral dilation of the lateral ventricles and the fourth ventricle.

The use of other techniques, such as positron emission tomography and nuclear magnetic resonance, have also revealed evidence of brain pathology in autistic subjects without focusing attention on a particular brain area.

More relevant data concern some alterations of the cerebellum and the limbic system, with particular reference to the amygdala and the hippocampus. The neuronal cells in these areas are smaller than normal and their density is excessive. In the limbic system, there is an area called the amygdala, known as able to regulate aspects of social and emotional behavior.

A study of high-functioning autistic children showed that their amygdala showed qualitative impairments but that another area of the brain, the hippocampus, did not present them at all. Muds on the behavior of some monkeys with amygdala destroyed by birth have shown that growing up, like autistic children, they became increasingly closed in themselves and showed a tendency to avoid social contacts.

The hippocampus is, instead, implicated in learning and memory. Children with autism would find it difficult to connect new information with information already stored because damage to the hippocampus interferes with the ability to maintain information in memory. In fact, studies on animals with lesions or removal of the hippocampus would exhibit stereotyped behaviors, self-stimulators and hyperactivity.

The cerebellum is one of the most active centers of the brain and Purkinje cells are critical elements in its data integration system. The scarcity of Purkinje cells in the cerebellum of autistic children shows how without these cells the cerebellum is incapable of doing its job, that is, receiving information about the outside world, calculating its meaning and preparing other areas of the brain to respond appropriately. Courchesne and his collaborators, with images obtained thanks to magnetic resonance, have highlighted cerebellum atrophy due to a lack of development within the uterus of the lobes VI and VII. Those with autism need more time than normal to shift attention, and the VI and VII lobes could play a decisive role in this regard.

From more in-depth research, the cerebellum would also seem to be involved in other processes such as verbalization, learning, attention and the emotional dimension.

## Neurotransmitters

Neurotransmitters, the chemical messengers of the central nervous system, play a role of primary importance in the cognitive, emotional and behavioral dimensions. The neurotransmitters involved in autism research are manifold and the brain sites of the alterations concern the whole brain area: from the frontal lobes, to the amygdala, to the hippocampus, to the ventricles, to the corpus callosum. The investigation of neurotransmitter systems has highlighted alterations in the metabolism of serotonin and, in particular, high serotonin levels in the blood of some autistic subjects in their entirety, with abnormalities of platelet uptake and release correlation at the intellectual level and age of subjects.

For some authors autism would be associated with dopamine deficiency; inadequate functioning of the dopaminergic system could justify some of the main symptoms of autism. The main activity of dopamine is, in fact, to exercise control over the attentional, perceptive, communicative, motor, emotional and behavioral functions.

Furthermore, abnormalities of the endogenous opioid system have been documented, with their overproduction in the central nervous system of autistic subjects. These opioids would affect many aspects of life and the development process, inhibiting transmission in all the main neurotransmitter systems existing in the brain and influencing learning, perception, emotions and executive functions. Opioids may also be due to some alterations in the immune system in autism.

All these neurotransmitters are well represented in the amygdala, an important brain structure for aspects of social interaction.

Recently, altered levels of oxytocin in the blood and spinal fluid have given this peptide a role in the pathogenesis of some autistic behaviors.

In conclusion, each of the data reported so far is present in some children and absent in others; therefore, these data, globally considered, cannot be included in a unitary interpretative model.

## Causal factors

The causal or etiological factors refer to the causes capable of altering the neurobiological pattern underlying the mental functioning which ultimately results in the autistic behavioral framework.

In general, two types of etiological factors are considered:

- genetic factors;

- acquired factors.

Genetic factors are the factors most implicated in the etiology of infantile autism, as shown by studies conducted on siblings of autistic children and on pairs of twins, one of which was diagnosed as autistic.

In siblings of children with infantile autism the incidence of the disorder would be about 2%; a risk with a frequency from 50 to 100 times higher than that estimated in the general population, moreover, the siblings of people with autism are significantly more exposed to mental retardation, speech disorders, and socialization. Regardless of the presence of a defined autistic situation, ascendants and collaterals tend to share cognitive-behavioral and language alterations in an attenuated form, which in some members may precipitate and determine the characteristic behavioral phenotype.

In 1997 Folstein and Rutter, in a study conducted on twenty-two pairs of twins, eleven monozygotic and ten heterozygotes, one of whom was diagnosed as autistic, confirmed the importance of genetic factors in determining autism. In particular, a concordance between monozygotic twins ranging from 86% to 92% was reported; while, in the heterozygous twins the concordance would be about 26% with the presence, moreover, of intellectual deficits and language disorders.

Some genetically inherited pathological conditions such as fragile X syndrome, tuberous sclerosis, neurofibromatosis, and phenylketonuria often occur in comorbidity with autism. However, these associations are not the rule and the strongest evidence emerging from the research is that the autism gene does not exist; genetic alterations can be considered as an important component of the multifactorial etiology of autism.

The acquired factors are those attributable to pre-, peri- or post-natal noxae, such as intrauterine infections, hypoxia in labor, immediate postpartum asphyxia.

These conditions can interfere with brain development and have long-term effects on the child's mental, sensory, linguistic and social functions. However, at present, there is no significant association between one of such pathogenic noxae and autistic disorder.

## Diagnosis guidelines

Autism is a very complex behavioral disorder and includes a wide variety of symptoms that typically occur before the child is three years old.

However, different modalities of onset of autistic symptomatology are detected; in some children, it is present from the first year of life, in others it is evident starting from the second year, through a sharp regression or a progressive slowing of the pace of development, in others, it is characterized by a fluctuating trend.

The concept of autism has undergone significant changes over the course of half a century, such as the transition from a single syndrome, which could vary along a continuum of increasing gravity to a spectrum of disorders characterized by very different and associated clinical manifestations in various ways.

In the subsequent classifications to that of Kanner we can see the attempt to break free from its classification and thus abandon the conception that sees autism inserted in the group of schizophrenia.

In 1980, in the third edition of the Diagnostic and Statistical Manual of Mental Disorders (DSM-III), the change in perception of autism is realized with the introduction of the chapter dedicated to Generalized Developmental Disorders and with the definitive abandonment of the concept of autism as infantile psychosis (DSM-II, 1968).

Autism, as a generalized disorder, involves diffuse aspects of the personality, such as perceptual development, attention, motor skills, cognitive abilities, language, imitation and environmental adaptation.

In the new international classification drafted by the World Health Organization (WHO), autism is included in neurobiological developmental disorders, with a strong organic component deduced from the presence of a genetic concordance greater than 50%.

Autism is currently recognized as one of the Pervasive or Generalized Developmental Disorders (DPS).

The etiology is still not known about the autistic disorder, therefore the only diagnostic criteria are based on behavioral indicators defined by the Diagnostic and Statistical Manual of Mental Disorders (DSM-VI) written by the American Psychiatric Association, and by the International Classification of Diseases (ICD-10) drafted by the World Health Organization.

In the fourth edition of the DSM the most important novelty, compared to the previous edition (DSM III-R, 1987), is the displacement of the category to which autism belongs, Generalized Developmental Disorders, from Axis II characterized by disorders at the end long, stable and with poor prognosis to Axis I with episodic and transient disorders. This means having recognized that the symptoms of autism can vary and diminish. Furthermore, in DSM-IV a further autistic condition is introduced which is called Asperger's disorder.

In children with this pathology autistic behavior is observed around three or four years, after a period in which psychomotor development, language development and intellectual level are substantially adequate. In this disorder, what becomes more and more compromised is the capacity for social relationships and the variety of social interests. Intelligence, on the other hand, is almost normal.

Children with Asperger's disorder, like children with autistic disorder, lack the development of what has been called the theory of the mind.

Currently, the Diagnostic and Statistical Manual of Mental Disorders-Text Revision (DSM-IV-TR) is the most widely used internationally.

The criteria with diagnostic meaning are represented by:

- qualitative impairment of social interaction;

- qualitative impairment of verbal and non-verbal communication;

- modalities of behavior, narrow, repetitive and stereotyped interests and activities.

The definition of autism contained within the WHO classification (ICD-10) is very similar to that given by DSM-IV-TR, in this case we speak of childish autism and not of childhood disorder.

In ICD-10 the description of the atypical autism framework that is differentiated from infantile autism is interesting.

In atypical autism, although there is an impairment of development, anomalies in social interaction and communication and stereotypes of behavior, these are also evident after three years - atypical in the age of onset - or, even, highlighting before three years, do not entirely satisfy the three groups of main symptoms - atypicality in the symptomatology -.

**Table 1.1. Diagnostic criteria for autistic disorder (DSM – IV-TRTR):**

| |
|---|
| (1). **A total of 6 (or more) items from (1), (2), and (3), with at least 2 from (1), and one each from (2) and (3):** |

(1). qualitative impairment of social interaction, manifested with at least 2 of the following:

    i)   marked impairment in the use of various non-verbal behaviors, such as direct gaze, mimic expression, body postures, and gestures, which regulate social interaction.

    ii)  inability to develop relationships with peers appropriate to the level of development.

    iii) lack of spontaneous search for the sharing of joys, interests or goals with other people (eg, not showing, bringing, or calling attention to objects of personal interest).

    iv) lack of social or emotional reciprocity;

(2). qualitative impairment of the communication as expressed by at least 1 of the following:

    i)   delay or total lack of the development of the spoken language (not accompanied by an attempt to compensate through alternative methods of communication such as gestures or mimicry).

    ii)  in subjects with adequate language, marked impairment of the ability to initiate or sustain a conversation with others.

    iii) use of stereotyped and repetitive language or eccentric language.

    iv) lack of various and spontaneous simulation games, or games of social imitation appropriate to the level of development;

(3). restricted, repetitive and stereotyped behavior, interests and activities, as expressed by at least one of the following:

    i)   absorbing dedication to one or more types of

narrow and abnormal stereotyped interests or by intensity or by focus.

ii) completely rigid submission to unnecessary habits or specific rituals.

iii) stereotyped and repetitive motor mannerisms (beating or twisting hands or the head, or complex, movements of the whole body).

iv) persistent and excessive interest in parts of objects;

(2). **Delays or abnormal functioning in at least one of the following areas, with onset before 3 years of age:**

(1). social interaction,

(2). the language used in social communication.

(3). symbolic game or imagination.

(3). **The anomaly is not better attributable to Rett's Disorder or Childhood Disintegrative Disorder.**

## Comorbidity with other disorders

From an exclusively clinical-descriptive point of view the fundamental nucleus of the autistic disorder can occur in different patients with considerable variations in the degree of clinical expressiveness. Moreover, alongside the basic disorder, a series of characteristic symptoms and associated disorders such as mental retardation and epilepsy manifest themselves in a variable way.

## Mental delay

The relationship between mental retardation and autism has been and is the cause of heated debates.

In the past a source of confusion has been the tendency to consider autism a pure disorder, that is that it is not found in the presence of other syndromes, such as mental retardation.

Tager-Flusberg and Baron-Choen believe that the category of high-functioning autism is used to distinguish this pure form of autism from that related to mental retardation.

Currently, mental retardation and autism are considered as two independent disorders, nevertheless, it has become a clinical practice to find the presence of both and it is clear that there is a close relationship between them. Most autistic subjects, around 75% of cases, have varying degrees of mental retardation and just over 10% have normal or rarely superior mental abilities. Both in subjects with delay and those with normal intelligence, the performance profile is often inhomogeneous with the presence of areas of great skill such as memory, calculation, spatial skills and deeply compromised areas. The overall clinical picture is strongly conditioned by the extent of cognitive impairment.

They are very often associated in the most serious conditions with striking behavioral alterations, such as hyperactivity, self and/or hetero aggressiveness; the mood is very changeable, with rapid and unpredictable fluctuations from flattening and apathy to the excitement. The high presence of mental retardation does not necessarily imply a neurological origin of all those who are affected; on the theoretical level, it is, in fact, possible to argue that even very early depressive or bipolar disorders can have a disruptive effect on mental growth and thus lead to a delay. Furthermore, having ascertained that at least 10% of medium-serious delays are due to an anomaly in the number or structure of chromosomes, would explain the genetic origin of some cases of mental retardation or autism.

# Epilepsy

Epilepsy is a fairly common disorder in autism spectrum disorders.

The rate of comorbidity varies between 30-40% of cases, depending on the age and type of disorder.

Already in Kanner's early descriptions, in a population of people with autism, epilepsy occurred in 5-30% of cases, against the value of 0.5% of the general population of children and adolescents. The two most risky moments of onset of epileptic manifestations of those suffering from autism are early childhood and adolescence. In early childhood epilepsy occurs in a third of cases with frequent myoclonic seizures that can determine, by themselves, the conditions for the development of autistic symptoms. Infantile spasms with hypsarithmia are selectively associated with autism, as evidenced by a classic Finnish study of Riikonen and Amnell of 1981, which found them in 16% of cases. Often this form of epilepsy is linked to neuropathological alterations such as tuberous sclerosis and congenital disorders of neuronal migration which, in turn, are often connected with autism.

Complex partial seizures and generalized tonic-clonic seizures generally arise in adolescence, while the small evil is rare.

"The age of onset, the characteristics and the evolution of epileptic seizures depend more on the severity of the underlying brain damage than on autism itself." A lesion affecting the temporal lobe, for example, may represent the disturbing element in the development of social competences or an epileptogenic focus responsible for comitial symptoms.

# Chapter II MUSICOTHERAPY

## 2.1 Definitions and principles

Explaining what music therapy is is not easy because of the vast number of definitions formulated within the scientific landscape; it is also a relatively young discipline and still in progress.

Rolando Benenzon, an Argentine neurologist and psychotherapist, one of the pioneers of music therapy, laments the lack of a real theoretical paradigm for this discipline, halfway between psychotherapy and a science.

It is interesting to note first of all that the concept of music is conceived in the widest form of sound intended, in turn, as a primordial acoustic entity that interacts in the psychobiological relationship with a man. In this relationship, different factors come into relationship, not only organized and structured music, therefore, but all sound stimuli of any nature and the relative sources; propagation systems for sound and reception stimuli; the acoustic reception of the nervous system; the psychobiological reaction and the elaboration of the answer.

The reflection on the therapeutic function of sound is today so developed that it even seems difficult to define music therapy in a unified way. In general, we can try to think of it as the science that reflects on the relationship of biological and psychological nature between sound and human beings and consequently elaborates strategies to maintain, improve, restore the mental and physical health of the subjects who have emotional, physical, mental and psychological handicaps.

Today for Benenzon a definition of music therapy according to its own experience could be: "music therapy is a psychotherapeutic technique, which uses sound, music, movement, and musical instruments to determine a historical process of constraint, between the therapist and his patient or a group of patients, to improve the quality of life and rehabilitate and recovering patients for society "

Music can be used to get in touch with various aspects of the human being, aspects related to motor incoordination and physical problems, aspects related to the psychic sphere and aspects related to the emotional sphere. But music becomes a valid instrument even when working in social recovery, in all those forms of social distress where through the use of a non-verbal language it is possible to recreate a dialogue.

Music is often used as a background in various types of therapy, with different purposes related to the type of work performed, but it becomes music therapy only when it is the stimulus and the carrier vehicle from which an artistic-therapeutic work starts, for this it is an art therapy with links to all other artistic-expressive forms.

It is clear how much music is a very broad concept within the music therapy context.

*"Music is the art of organizing sounds over time".*

It is a non-verbal language, capable of stimulating the senses and arousing emotions and feelings. "... Music therapy is both an art, a science, and an interpersonal process. As an art, it is linked to subjectivity, creativity, and beauty. As a science it is linked to objectivity, the community, reproducibility and truth. As an interpersonal process, it is linked to empathy, intimacy, communication, mutual influence, and role relationship ".

In 1996 the World Music Therapy Federation gave the following definition: "Music therapy is the use of music and/or musical elements (sound, rhythm, melody, and harmony) by a qualified music therapist, with a user or a group, in a process aimed at facilitating and encouraging communication, relationship, learning, motor skills, expression, organization, and other relevant therapeutic objectives to satisfy physical, emotional, mental, social and cognitive needs.

Music therapy aims to develop the individual's potential and/or residual functions in such a way that they can better achieve Intra and interpersonal integration and consequently improve the quality of life thanks to a preventive, rehabilitative or therapeutic process ".

It is useful to understand what music therapy consists of, and to orientate oneself in its variegated world, is to know how it is used and by whom.

## 2.2 Background

Music therapy has ancient roots. Even before someone gave her this name, there were already those who consciously used music to relieve pain or psychological suffering.Music has accompanied the whole history of man and there are many documents that, through time and space, bear witness to it.

Once upon a time the sound was given particular importance believing that it was a cosmic force, present since the origins of the world and that it had taken the verbal form.

Among primitive men, there was the belief that every being, living or dead, possessed a secret personal sound to which he had to respond and which made him vulnerable to magic. For this reason some magic rituals attempted to discover the sound to which the patient or the spirit who lived in it responded.

The healing properties of music were already known to the ancients and indications are found in history, mythology, and philosophy.

The first paper concerning music therapy or referring to the healing power of music is in the Bible: "... *and so, whenever the bad spirit that came from God came upon Saul, David took the harp and began to play; Saul calmed down and was better because the evil spirit withdrew from him and left him in peace* ".

In classical Greece and ancient Rome music was used in a reasoned and logical way, without magical or religious implications, but with the ability to stick exclusively to the clinical situation and be applied in the prevention and treatment of physical and mental illnesses.

Plato and Aristotle could be considered the precursors of music therapists. Aristotle spoke of the authentic medical value of music in uncontrolled emotions and attributed to it a beneficial effect at the level of catharsis.

Plato boasted the music and the dance for the fears and the phobic anxieties: "... the music was not given to the man only to flatter his senses, but also to calm the torments of the soul and the movements that a body tempts full of imperfections ".

Plato in the Republic attributed to music the power to shape the soul and the body. According to this conception, therefore, music had the faculty of forming, transforming, modifying the body and the spirit. This is the concept that we find, albeit in a different context, in the music therapy paradigm understood as an organized sound event, inserted in a precise relational framework, capable of bringing about change in the subjects involved according to therapeutic values.

Pythagoras called music musical medicine and used it to quell madness.

Celio Aureliano tells that the ancients treated painful parts of the body with the influence of sound, especially if they sang on those parts so that the shudder resulting from the percussion of the air brought them relief.

During the Middle Ages there was a wide appeal to music and in some medieval texts, it is told how musicians brought relief to the suffering of the sick in the hospital and how the magical properties of music were also transmitted to musical instruments. From the finds found, today it can be affirmed that the man built the first musical instruments more than thirty-five thousand years ago.

In the eighteenth century, it was preferred to talk about the effects of music on the body's fibers. Thanks to a mechanical effect, the regular musical vibrations re-establish the harmony of the fibers; the stretched fibers spread out little by little and the music distracts the patient's soul from his sad worries, forcing him to take an interest in something other than his illness.

Tissot made a difference between stimulating and calming music that makes the patient forget the indisposition even if he is not able to suppress the cause of the illness.

Today the idea of music as a magical and thaumaturgical event has been replaced by a new concept closer to modern science, that of music therapy.

The use of music therapy as a methodology and as a professional tool is extremely ancient, in fact, as much as the existence of music itself. His development began when the power and influence of music on the emotional-affective dimension experimented for the first time.

Music therapy began to outline the first lines of discipline, starting in 1811 thanks to the work of Pietro Lichtnenthal, an Italian-Hungarian physician and composer, who wrote the treatise on "Influence of music on the human body".

Since then, almost two centuries have passed and today music therapy has become a complex discipline from a theoretical point of view that addresses different fields of application.

The real scientific researches on the physiological changes induced by music through the measurement of its effects on respiration, heart rate, circulation and blood pressure date back to the last century. Music acts on the neurovegetative system that regulates body functions such as transpiration, heart rhythm, blood pressure and facilitates the release of everyone's emotions and creative resources. The approach to the person is holistic in an inseparable unity of mind and body.

In 1950, with the foundation in the United States of the National Association for Music Therapy, the birth of music therapy as a scientific methodology officially falls. From 1953, the minimum educational and clinical training requirements necessary to become music therapists were established in the music therapy programs of the various universities.

Since that time, in all countries of the world, various music therapy associations have been founded that stand out in national associations, such as AIM in Italy, with representatives in international associations, such as the European Music Therapy in Europe, which make all refer to a world association of music therapy, the World Federation of Music Therapy.

The attempts to integrate music with therapeutic activity are part of human history, we can say that they are inherent in its nature; the voices, sounds, and movements that accompanied him in the ancient rituals of healing became and evolved with the man himself, in a continuous search for support and help in the difficult moments of existence.

Today, music therapy means above all using sound, music and movement to improve communication with the outside or to get some particular therapeutic benefits in categories of subjects such as autistic children or those with communication problems, sensory disabilities or mental retardation and adults with dementia or neurodegenerative diseases.

## 2.3. The figure of the music therapist

The music therapist is the one who knows how to manage the listening and the expression of the codes of non-verbal communication; consequently, it must develop its analog capabilities to the maximum. The music therapist is also the one who manages the session, who gives the deliveries and who relates directly with the patient. In music therapy the word during a session is a sound. The music therapist often describes singing the actions performed by the patient; the word is not necessary, the nodal point of the session is to express itself creatively through music. Acting in music therapy makes sense in knowing sound like a relationship, the original relationship is woven into life before being born, the relationship with the world, with others, with oneself where the sound is the vibratory wave that testifies to life. For the music therapist, the first musical instrument is the human body, it is the first orchestra is that of the sounds we hear in the maternal uterus; music therapy seeks the musicality of these sounds and in a certain sense teaches us that we must return to dialogue even without words, like when we were in the womb.

Sound from childhood, in the mother-child relationship, is communication and dialogue and is at the same time intermediary in the music therapist-patient relationship.

"The typical relationship we refer to is the primary mother-child relationship; it constitutes the model for the therapeutic relationship, through which the entire tuning work can be performed ". Through a work based on deeply participated empathic interaction processes, which we call attunements, it, therefore, becomes possible to facilitate both verbal and non-verbal communication, the quality of learning and affective availability.

The goal should be to bring patients as close as possible to what they are, giving them the space to express themselves and the perception of feeling welcomed for what they really are. Hence the difficulty in tuning in with the severe handicap. This difficulty, which at first sight is unsurpassed and unsolvable, is feasible if the music therapist, with an effort to decode, can interpret at first sight incomprehensible needs, just as happens in the early tuning of mothers with their children. Infants, in fact, do not have an articulated language and only with crying can they communicate their every need. The task of the music therapist dealing with the severe handicap is exactly the same, he must seek a channel of attunement with the main mode of behavior of the patient.

The area in which it will search for this tuning channel is non-verbal communication.

Music therapy intends to offer the possibility of opening new channels of communication and expression to those people for whom verbal communication is limited or impossible.

The music therapist, therefore, deals with the intentional construction of communicative relationships for therapeutic purposes, through the use of two distinct elements:

the relationship: for the development of which one can make use of musical activities and other expressive practices;

 music: through which to realize a form of non-verbal communication

Both the music and the report are integral parts of the music therapy meeting.

The most significant relationships in music therapy are a patient-music and patient-music therapist. However, it must be emphasized that depending on the orientation of the music therapist these two relationships assume different weights.

If music is used as a therapy, the music therapist leaves the main role of music and the patient-music relationship becomes the primary agent of therapeutic change. If instead, music is used in therapy, the patient-music therapist relationship is put in the foreground and becomes almost a more interpersonal than musical relationship.

Patients and music therapists both bring something of themselves into play and their personalities are deeply involved in the therapeutic process.

The authentic relationship is one in which the patient relates to the music or the music therapist for what they are and for what they offer in the present. By creating a success-oriented atmosphere without threats, establishing a relationship with the patient to promote growth and structuring the environment to help the patient achieve certain therapeutic goals, the music therapist transforms a simple musical activity into music therapy.

During a music therapy meeting, when the evolution of the situation or a transformation is generated through an action, a sound or a movement, what changes are not only the bodily or musical parameters but also and above all the relational parameters. The relation parameter is, therefore, the synthesis parameter that includes and brings together all the other indicators such as gaze, posture, and movement, rhythmic behavior, voice, instruments, and communication.

The most recent definition disclosed by the APMT dictates "music therapy provides a framework in which a mutual relationship can be established between the client and the therapist.

The development of the relationship allows changes to take place, both in the condition of the client and in the form taken by the therapy [...]. Using music with creativity in a clinical setting, the music therapist tries to establish interaction, a shared musical experience, aiming to achieve therapeutic goals ".

A therapist is, by definition, an expert who uses the principles of personal and professional ethics to conduct his work with clients. In music therapy these principles concern issues such as musical and clinical competence, professional conduct, customer rights, research.

How long is the road through which a handicap is produced by a neurological, sensorial or psychic deficit, just as long as the path that a music therapist must first form and then put him in a position to develop an operational strategy aimed at attuning the handicap? In reality, if it is true that, in the words of Seneca, art is long and life is short and therefore learning a profession well is always not a simple matter, this is all the more true for professions that have to do with the relationship and with the handicap since they require to face a non-linear and complex path.

## Active and receptive music therapy: the intervention techniques used

Music therapy is an ancient therapy, if not the oldest. From the Greeks, we know that they distinguished active and passive music therapy and its application in homeopathy and allopathy.

Music therapy differs from other treatment therapies in that it relies heavily on musical experience as an agent, a context or a catalyst for a therapeutic experience.

In therapy the musical experience must be conceived both from an active and a receptive point of view. The modalities of music therapy interventions are traditionally divided into two main types:

active music therapy: refers to a methodology in which the music therapist and the patient interact with each other improvising, that is, producing sounds directly with the use of musical instruments, with the voice or with one's own body and influencing each other. The musical instruments that are used are easy to approach and do not require preliminary knowledge; the body is the basic toolbox through which one moves in the awareness of one's own rhythmic and sound potentials in attunement with the self. Active music therapy establishes non-verbal communication between music therapists and patients based on trust.

Once confidence is obtained, we proceed by applying the mirroring technique in which the music therapist imitates the sounds, follows the movements, the patient's expressions to strengthen the emotional bond; subsequently, the technique of variation and re-elaboration of the sound material is applied to induce the patient to change and to enrich expression and communication.

Active psychomusical techniques are considered to be authentic psychotherapeutic methods whose aim is the exploration of the internal world of the individual, the mobilization of energies and psychic dynamics and the reconstruction and reorganization of the inner life, to accept himself, others and reality of its becoming.

receptive music therapy: it is based on listening to sounds and music chosen by the music therapist and given to the patient life or with audio techniques. The patient is left with the autonomy of perception, imagination, and elaboration related to the proposed music. Receptive music therapy is fundamentally based on the observation that listening to sounds and music allows the patient to relax, to feel emotions, to evoke positive memories and to stimulate the production of mental images to explore the inside of the consciousness to change the physical conditions, emotional, intellectual and relational. Sound stimuli allow the release of neurotransmitters and neuromodulators that modulate the behavior and affectivity of human beings.

Their concentration changes in each individual when listening to their music. The vibrations picked up by the inner ear, penetrating at various depths, cause transformations in the electrobiochemical processes within the mind and the organism through which one enters into vibration when it vibrates on the same wavelength of sound. Listening to music, which includes musical experiences of all kinds, must be considered an integral part of music therapy. Treatment with receptive music therapy is particularly favorable if applied in cases of neuropsychological diseases.

Active and receptive music therapy can be proposed in individual or group settings.

Each type of musical experience, both active and receptive, has its own unique therapeutic applications and benefits; therefore, limiting music therapy by excluding any of these experiences means depriving the patient of part of the resources of the discipline. In any case, the needs of the patient must take precedence over the positions or preferences of the music therapist.

## Principles of music therapy

Music therapy as a methodology and technique of clinical application is based on the following principles:

- the principle of ISO,

- the intermediary object,

- the integrator object.

These principles are not the exclusive prerogative of music therapy since they can be the basis of other non-verbal clinical techniques. However, they assume, in music therapy, particular characteristics that distinguish them.

The reference model is that proposed by the Argentine neurologist and psychotherapist Rolando Benenzon, considered one of the leading experts in the world of the application of music therapy in cases of autism, of patients in a coma and Alzheimer's disease.

This model is based not so much on the production of music by the patient but on the relationship between patient and music therapist, which is facilitated by the presence of sounds or musical instruments.

## The principle of ISO

The basic idea is that each of us has our own sound or ISO identity, composed of all those sounds and rhythms that have accompanied our lives, from conception to the present. The ISO is an element that characterizes each individual and is made up of the sum of the intra-uterine sound experience linked to internal perceptions and to that of birth, the fruit of external perceptions.

This biological time derived from the speed of gait, heart rate, and breathing is unique for each of us, is structured over time and is in perpetual movement. The term ISO means equal and alludes to a sound identity to be sought; in fact, it is the music therapist's task to identify the mental time of the patient to accord him a certain sound or musical time, intending to open a communication channel through which to operate than the recovery.

For Benenzon the ISO is "a sound mosaic that is structured over time", the concept of the mosaic is more clear and takes on a double connotation with the description that the author proposes of four types of ISO: a universal ISO, a gestalt ISO, a complementary ISO, and a group ISO.

The universal ISO is the dynamic sound identity that characterizes or identifies all human beings, regardless of the particular social, cultural, historical and psycho-physiological context. It can be traced back to the thread and ontogenetic heritage of humanity, it includes the sonorities related to the heartbeat, to the processes of inhalation and exhalation, to the intestinal noises, to the voice of the mother at the moment of birth and in the first days of life, as well as to the sounds of nature, such as that produced by wind and water, and again, childhood melodies and lullabies.

Everything that makes up the universal ISO is fertile ground on which to build the relationship and lay the foundations for encouraging the emergence of any communication process.

The gestalt ISO is grafted onto the sound prototypes of the universal ISO. During the months of gestation, it receives stimuli from three major sources that will favor its structuring.

From the outside, through the amniotic fluid: the voice of the father and other voices, noises of the social environment, musical-cultural sounds, unidentifiable vibrations, various types of acoustic phenomena.

From inside the mother: the voice of the mother, rhythm of inspiration and exhalation, heartbeat, the crunch of the uterine walls, joint and muscle sounds, sounds typical of the overall functioning of the organism, gravitational movements and other unidentifiable phenomena.

From the same body of the fetus: the blood flow with all its characteristics of nutrition, respiration, thermoregulation, vital functions, the heartbeat, the sound phenomena of the functioning of his organism.

The gestalt ISO allows to discover the communication channel par excellence of the subject and is strongly connected with the unique and unrepeatable history of every single person. The gestalt ISO takes its name from Gestalt psychology which invites us to consider the original perception.

Each individual organizes any perceived sound-musical element against the background of his own inner life and experiences, filling it with a very special, personal, subjective and intimate meaning. The subject does not perceive a set of elementary sounds, but a global sensation. All that we hear, perceive, live and everything that has been handed down to us for generations remains written in us, is the memory of our body. For this reason, when referring to the emergence of the child's basic rhythmicity, it means helping him to become aware of the spontaneous musicality that is already part of him.

The complementary ISO is made up of the minimal variations of the gestalt ISO that occur under the influence of particular environmental conditions.

The group ISO reflects the social pattern within which the individual evolves. It depends on the work carried out over time by the groups in which the gestalt ISOs of each individual adapt, intertwining with each other to constitute a creative identity proper to the group in question.

The ISO of each group has a particular biological time because a determined logic, rhythms, forms, sequences, and cadences that characterize it are established and structured. The group ISO is a dynamic that pervades the group as a synthesis of all sound identities and gathers within itself a set of psycho-physiological factors, sounds and movements that depend on the gestalt ISO of each individual.

The group ISO is fundamental in order to reach an integration unit within a therapeutic group in a non-verbal context.

The concept of group ISO is expanded, in an ethnomusicological perspective, anthropological and music therapeutic, to that of cultural ISO. "Cultural ISO is the product of the global cultural configuration of which the individual and his group are a part. It is the sound identity of a relatively homogeneous cultural community ".

Benenzon believes that the group ISO, due to its characteristics, leads to the concept of ethnic identity, a set, that is, of heterogeneous cultural groups that express themselves through their own sounds. Ethnic identity cannot be separated from the sound identity that each individual possesses as belonging to a specific cultural community. This sound cultural identity develops and is enriched based on the processes of learning of one's own culture and based on the rules that govern it.

In conclusion, Benenzon states that the gestalt ISO and the complementary ISO operate on an individual level based on physiological and musical development factors; the ISO group and the cultural ISO, on the other hand, operate on a collective level in relation to social-cultural factors. It is however evident that elements of the gestalt ISO of each individual flow into the group ISO and into the cultural ISO.

**The intermediary object**

The intermediary object is the second fundamental principle on which music therapy is articulated. The principle of the intermediary object derives from the concept of Winnicott's transitional object and refers to every element capable of allowing the passage of communicative energy from one individual to another. The intermediary object has, precisely, the purpose of thinning the communication channels. The mother's body is the first intermediary object of communication, after which the elements that will be the extension of this body will follow, but also the father brings intermediary objects of communication in the relationship.

It was J.G. Rojas Bermudez to use the term intermediate object first in psychodrama; with the use of puppets, he was able to create bonds that allowed the patient to get out of his isolation and then enter into a relationship with the auxiliary self.

I also note that the marionette as an emitting source, devoid of human characteristics, was considered by the patient an inoffensive object and therefore therapeutically usable.

An intermediary object can be defined as the communication tool capable of acting therapeutically on the patient within the relationship, without giving rise to states of intense alarm; it has the following characteristics:

- real and concrete existence;

- harmlessness: it does not give life by itself to alarm reactions:

- malleability: it can be used at will for any role;

- it is a transmitter: it allows communication replacing the physical bond and maintaining the distance between the partners;

- adaptability: adapted to the needs of the subject;

- it is similar to oneself: it allows a very intimate relationship, as the subject can identify him with himself;

- it is instrumental: it can be used as an extension of the subject;

- it is identifiable: it can be recognized immediately.

For Benenzon musical instruments and sound, or the sounds they emit, can be considered intermediary objects and possess all the characteristics stated above. There is however a difference between the puppet, as an intermediary object, and the musical instruments. A marionette is a lifeless object, in it the source of sound emission derives directly from the psychodrammist; the relationship, therefore, with the human source will be very narrow.

The musical instrument, on the other hand, has the source of sound emission that characterizes it and it is owned independently of the music therapist. A musical instrument lends itself well to the role of the intermediary object in that it possesses properties, sonority, the form that affect the gestalt ISO and, to a lesser extent, the universal and complementary ISO by creating extrapsychic channels of communication and opening up sclerotic and stereotyped ones.

Intermediate instruments are not only the musical instruments, conventional and not, used in the setting, but also the body, including that of the therapist, can represent an important channel of communication.

The body is the most complete musical instrument in every respect. It is, in fact, at the origin of musical instruments since the latter is simply an extension of the human body. The body, however, does not meet all the conditions required by the intermediary object since it can awaken anxiety and alarm situations. At the beginning, in fact, the use must be done at a distance, to avoid the melee that in some patients can cause escape or panic.

Benenson's goal is to stimulate a possible patient reaction in the patient-music therapist relationship through sound, acting on the sensory, motor and affective levels.

## The integrating object

The integrating object is considered the musical instrument that in a music therapy group prevails over the other instruments, becoming a leading tool able to concentrate and absorb the dynamics of the relationship between patient and music therapist.Integrating tools are simple, large-volume, rhythmic and powerful instruments of manipulation; facing outwards have clear sound possibilities.

They often belong to the class of membranophones, ie percussion instruments; the fundamentals are the drums, the bongos, the small timpani and the cymbals.The membranophones have the advantage of producing sounds not only by hitting them but also by caressing them, touching them, scratching them, thus opening up vast possibilities for sound, movement, and tactile sensations.

The drum is the ideal instrument especially at the beginning of the treatment and it is of fundamental importance since, like all membranophones with a resonance box, it reproduces the heartbeat and played standing up allows complete body movement.

The sound of the drum is powerful, pleasant and very primitive. Instruments such as the drum are called leading instruments because they combine the main characteristics required by music therapy, and they are generally chosen by the group's leading patients. Idiophones such as the xylophone, the rattles, the triangle, the marimbas are considered leading instruments from the melodic point of view. The xylophone, in particular, whose sound goes outwards, besides being melodic, causes a strong motor impulse.

In conclusion, clinical practice shows that the integrating object is connected to the group, cultural, complementary ISO and, to a lesser extent, to the gestalt ISO.

**Areas of intervention**

Music therapy is defined as "a discipline that uses the sonorous-musical element within the patient-operator relationship in a systematic intervention process with preventive, rehabilitative and therapeutic purposes".

The areas of music therapy intervention according to the purposes can be generalized to:

- educational-preventive field;

- habilitative-rehabilitative field;

- ambit (psycho) therapeutic.

The interventions must be adapted to the physical, emotional, social, spiritual needs of the patient-user.

Despite having a transdisciplinary nature, music therapy is a discipline of its own with its own well-defined characteristics that do not allow it to be confused with other treatment modalities.

The educational-preventive field pursues educational and possibly preventive aims towards the onset of relational diseases or social discomfort. This area concerns those interventions that use music to facilitate in individuals a path of knowledge and personal growth and to facilitate the development of subjective creativity allowing to give form to communicable and socializable expressive modalities within which to dissolve and transform potential pathogenic nuclei. The music in this area is used as a sound basis for the proposal of activities aimed at the development of knowledge and mastery of the body and movement, the main expression of individual personality and a fundamental means to relate with the environment and with others.

For the educational-preventive field, music therapy activities during pregnancy, childbirth, and birth accompanying are foreseen, for families with children up to thirty-six in absence of pathologies and in schools where music therapy is above all the means to promote the integration of the disabled and to encourage the harmonious development of all children. In the educational-preventive field, the music therapist can also work with the elderly, with adolescents from vulnerable social groups and with terminally ill patients.

The habilitative-rehabilitative field pursues rehabilitation purposes through methods and techniques related to the qualification-rehabilitation of the main psychophysical and social functions that regulate the good health of the individual. The object of the intervention of rehabilitation is not the disease in the first place, but what derives from the disease in terms of loss of functions.

Rehabilitation is a process of care from the outside, that is, rather than starting from the analysis of the pathogenic mechanisms that are the basis of a morbid event, the rehabilitation approach focuses on the prevention and recovery of complications.

The primary objective of music therapy in this field is to recover the capacities not directly involved with the type of deficit, skills that had developed normally before the morbid event; prevent, when possible, the transformation of the deficit into a handicap and stop or at least slow down its evolution.

It is a question of giving back to the subject a set of strategies aimed at increasing opportunities for the exchange of resources and affections and social and expressive abilities. The habilitative-rehabilitative intervention is different from a (psycho) therapeutic strategy from the inside while pursuing the same goal, that is, the patient's well-being.

The latter is implemented through the harmonization strategy, ie harmonizing parameters of the sonorous-musical type are respected, which respect the balance and general potential of the patient.

The rehabilitative intervention also requires large amounts of confidence, optimism, patience and encouragement that the operator profoundly and of which urges the expression on the part of patients.

Rehabilitation then becomes a strategy of stimulation and harmonization of those sensory, motor, cognitive, neuropsychological, psychic and social functions, indirectly involved in the process of disability formation, implemented through more or less specific techniques, but always from outside.

The techniques used range from vocal and instrumental practice exercises to analysis works and song compositions, to musical-theatrical dramatizations that can lead to the recovery of channels and the under-stimulated skills and the harmonious recomposition of the various parts of the individual.

For Kenneth Bruscia rehabilitative music therapy "is the use of musical experiences and relationships that are developed through them as a means to help clients, who have been debilitated by illness, injury or trauma, to regain as much as.

Rehabilitative music therapy interventions are aimed at functional recovery in neuromotor disorders such as Parkinson's disease, demyelinating syndromes, functional post-traumatic deficits, infantile cerebral palsy, muscular dystrophy and in sensory-perceptive pathologies such as blindness, deafness, deficiency of tactile and kinesthetic sensitivity and comatose syndromes.

In the habilitative-rehabilitative field, music therapy is also applied in cases of mental retardation and multi-handicap and the treatment of developmental and senile age disorders.In all areas, and in particular, in habilitation and rehabilitation, music therapy is part of an interdisciplinary, integrative and global rehabilitation perspective, where teamwork and collaboration between the various professional figures, families, local authorities and health and social care facilities are considered fundamental to offer users an effective and complete service.Music therapy due to its non-verbal language characteristics, depending on the type of context and relationship established, can act both in a rehabilitative sense and in a (psycho) therapeutic sense. However, since the terms rehabilitation and (psycho) therapy are distinct but not separable, music therapy, therefore, arises along a continuum that links these two areas of intervention. This appears all the more true in the context of the neuro-psychic handicap that is inserted in a context of strong social, preventive, rehabilitative and therapeutic significance.

The complexity of this handicap requires the formation of therapeutic-rehabilitative teams to which the music therapist belongs, which provides for the formulation and implementation of the therapeutic project. If the habilitative-rehabilitative intervention is a facilitative strategy from the outside of the cognitive-relational and socialization processes, the (psycho) therapeutic intervention is, instead, facilitation from within of the processes of self-awareness, of regulation of emotions and communication skills.In the (psycho) therapeutic field, the sonorous-musical element becomes a non-verbal communication channel that can favor the establishment of particular forms of interpersonal relationships.

In addition to musical experiences, verbal techniques are also frequently used and the patient-therapist relationship becomes the vehicle and condition of therapeutic change. Music therapy is one of the few activities offered to subjects with severe handicaps, it can generate a moment, even if of short duration, of well-being and relaxation. In the (psycho) therapeutic field, music therapy activities are aimed at the treatment of both particularly regressed subjects and non-evolved subjects in terms of object relation.

In situations of autism, childhood psychosis and adulthood music therapy represents, in fact, an extra-verbal communication channel that favors the expressiveness of the patient and the overcoming of situations of isolation. Thus, always in the (psycho) therapeutic field, in less compromised patients with personality and mood disorders, with psychoneuroses and somatoform disorders, music therapy can be a welcoming and restraining instrument capable of favoring the emergence of emotions and subjective experiences and then to act as an instrument of change in the internal world. The historical excursus and the areas of intervention have provided relevant data on the influence of music in multiple pathologies, this attributes a central role to music therapy, which must be considered a fundamental or adjuvant element for the stabilization of a state of well-being compatible with the framework clinical of the patient.

# Chapter III MUSICOTHERAPY AND AUTISM

*"Where the power of words stops, music begins ..."*

Music and communication The term communication is used in the biological, ecological, ethological and human fields to indicate an exchange of messages that can be implemented by single-celled organisms, animals, machines and human beings.

 While in the past only human verbal language was considered as a real language, from 1950 onwards it became common to define languages as other communication systems, human or otherwise, such as gestural-motor language, iconic language, language musical and animal language. In particular, music has a fundamental meaning in the history of human civilization, it is, in fact, capable of summarizing very important messages and meanings penetrating into human intimacy without problems of too many cultural or linguistic mediations.

The human being is characterized, in its essence, by communication, by the relationship with the other and with himself; a man who does not relate to anyone is unthinkable. Sometimes, however, this communication is complicated due to the lack of words or a language appropriate to what one wants to communicate, due to the presence of a language that cannot be understood by everyone or for the presence of psychic or physical deficits of the person.

Music, as a universal language, can eliminate some of these obstacles. Music, however, is not only communication with others, but becomes first of all communication with oneself; it favors the knowledge of oneself and one's own potential and makes it possible to integrate all the resources we have to live better. Music produces a predominantly emotional communication system, non-verbal or preverbal communication, and has great application precisely where verbal communication is not used and words become a barrier.

Music is one of the most significant means of communicating our personality, it can act through all the internal conditions, from the most superficial and insignificant to the most profound. Because of these characteristics, it is widely used and profoundly useful for the help of people with disabilities, and more specifically with children. For all people, but especially for communication disabilities, listening and making music means communicating.

Music is communication, or instrument of the fundamental relationship between oneself and others, between one's inner world and the surrounding environment.The musical sounds can involve all the senses through sound, visual, tactile and kinesthetic stimulations and offer the listener the possibility of answering through these same channels.

These multi-sensory aspects give the music a wide range of therapeutic possibilities.Music therapy is a subtle form of therapy, very appropriate for difficult children, such as non-communicants, valid where other therapies have not worked. Through music, the child finds a way to express himself that allows the therapist to establish relationships with him and to understand the deep feelings that the child does not want or cannot verbalize.

## Music therapy applied to autism

"One cannot communicate", this statement refers to inevitability, an essential characteristic of communication. Words or silence inevitably influence others who, either with silence or with words, postpone return messages thus giving rise to communication.

This transitive dynamic is not so obvious and obvious for the autistic child, its communicative channels, in fact, are often impenetrable and mysterious. The autistic child creates communication systems that are repeated continuously, giving rise to a series of stereotyped messages that Rolando Benenzon calls cysts of communication.

These rigid and repetitive forms of exchanges and messages form a protective shell that prevents the evolution of the child's communication and interpersonal relationships. In the autistic, incapable, to establish normal relations with others, music may be able to overcome the defensive barriers of the ego; in fact, it is said that every autistic life in an unbreakable glass cage; the music, however, can penetrate through the innumerable pores, invisible but still present in this cage. In this way, the music moves communication towards more elastic and less sterile forms and leads the child towards some communicative opening with the outside world.

Music therapy is, therefore, the first technique for approaching the human being, as is its application in infantile autism and is also the first technique for opening communication channels. Using predominantly non-verbal channels is extremely favorable for coming into contact with psychic structures and facilitating changes in a positive sense.

Therefore, music therapy aims at an approach, first sound, physical and psychic then, of the autistic child. Music therapy, where verbal communication is lacking, creates small breaches, minimal openings in the defensive system of the autistic child that seems to have the need to crystallize his inner world to defend himself from an external world that generates in him very strong anxious states. This crystallization also involves that part of the child that Benenzon calls sound or ISO identity. From a communicative point of view, the sound identity of the autistic child cannot be directly influenced by the sounds coming from the family and social environment; in this regard, music therapy could act as an intermediary and integrator between the child and the surrounding world. Music therapy certainly does not ensure either stable or definitive results alone, but it is a mediator of the communication between therapist and patient and, in some cases, it is the only one possible; with autistic children, it seems particularly useful because often it really succeeds in forcing its resistance and reducing the extent of the disorder of expression and communication.

## Benenzon's model in infantile autism

Rolando Benenzon, psychiatrist and music therapist, following his long personal experience with autistic children, describes the autistic condition as "a pathological and deformed extension of fetal psychism", in which the subject continues to reproduce behaviors similar to those of the fetus and, perceiving themselves thus in the intrauterine dimension, it tends to defend itself obstinately from the external world. It follows a marked tendency to isolation, a prediction for the covered places in which to find the protection, good contact with the water that reproduces the condition of the fetus immersed in the amniotic fluid, and with the sounds whose vibrations have already been perceived in the prenatal life stages.

Benenson's goal is, therefore, to work with a sort of fetus, which defends itself against the fears of an unknown external world and the feelings of lack of its internal world. In this situation it is particularly difficult to propose a bodily relationship, as there will be reactions of immediate rejection from contact, similar to the fetal reflex. Instead, the child's willingness to experience sound will make the musical intervention take on great importance to recreate alternative communication channels.

The opening of a communication channel with the autistic child seems to derive from the ability of sound and music to reactivate the modalities of archaic reactions still present in the child. To work with these children, in fact, it will be necessary to create environmental situations and stimuli that produce the reminiscence of the gestation period. The methodology described by Benenzon developed around the research of ISO and the intermediary object of the autistic child and involves three levels of work.

The first level is called the regression level: it is the model for listening to regressive sound proposals in order to produce in the patient, first of all, a regressive pleasure situation through listening to original sounds and, later, the opening of communication channels and the concurrent breakdown of defensive nodes.

In this context we find the research of ISO, that is, of the most significant regressive sounds for each child. During this phase the following sounds will be used:

- sounds belonging to the most primitive context, with strong regressive content, such as the heartbeat;

- inspiratory-expiratory sounds;

- bowel sounds;

- sounds of water;

the human voice that is used to emit simple even pleasurable noises such as whistling, popping the tongue, or as aggressive as grinding teeth, or provocative as grunting, rasping.

The recourse to even the slightest form of censorship could break that very subtle connection that the autistic child, in some topical moments, tries to construct with expressive modalities that upset the rigid relational dynamics. It is precisely these phases that must be managed by the music therapist with the desire to get involved until a profoundly uninhibited sound contact is established.

The transition from listening to the aforementioned regressive sounds to gradually more musical sounds will take place gradually. This step will serve to stimulate the slow but progressive transition to a state of pleasure in a context closer to reality.

The second level is called the communication level: during this phase the music therapist adopts a musical instrument, as an intermediary object, to reproduce the sound that touches the child's ego. In addition to the musical instrument, the body or objects of various kinds can also act as intermediary objects.

The music therapist working with the intermediary object and the found sound will establish a first encounter with the child who, in turn, communicates with the music therapist who uses the communication channels open at the first level, to enter as a human being.

The third level is the level of integration: in this last phase, also using the channels of the previous levels, the child communicates with the surrounding environment.

These sound moments can then be related to other techniques and means such as psychomotor skills. In fact, there is a close link between music and movement; they condition themselves like the key and the lock. Musical means often have the function of dissolving and motivating movement.

In autistic children we often see movements turned inwards: everything that should be destined to the outside and that derives from it is rejected. In this regard, Benenzon believes that it is useful to combine the sound stimulus with one or more movements, up to their coordination.

When this happens, it means that the patient is responding positively to stimulation, that there is a relationship between the child and the outside world and that the message from the outside has penetrated the barrier that surrounds the autistic child.

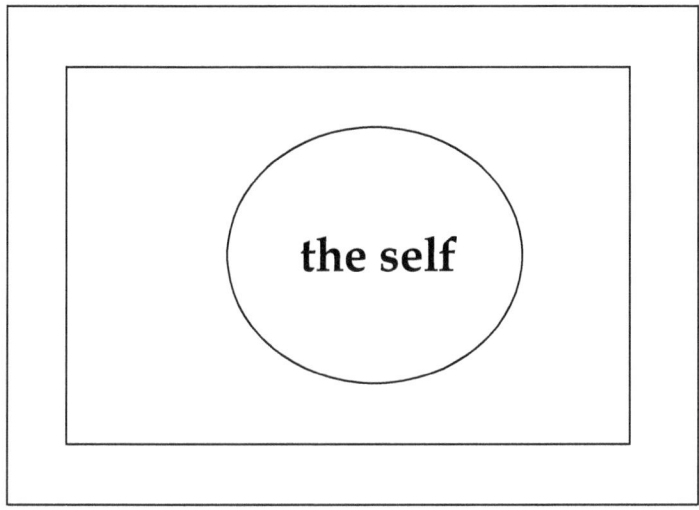

Fig. 3.1. Autistic child

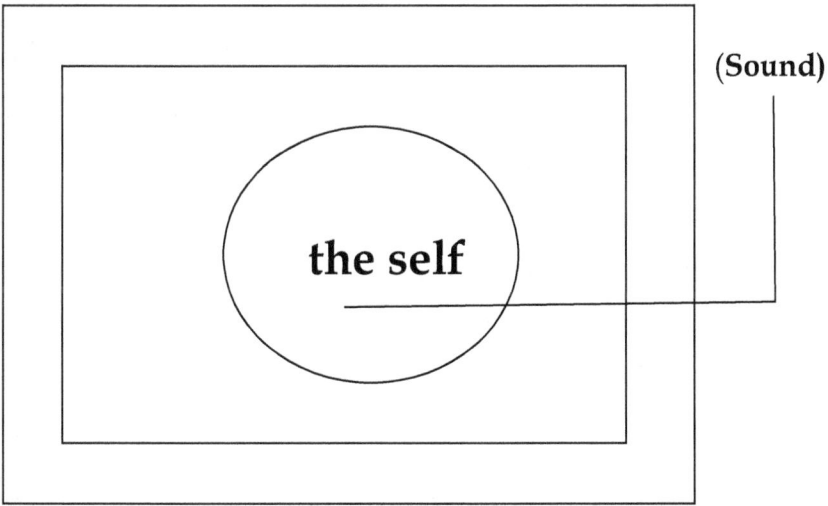

Fig. 3.2. The first approach

Fig. 3.1. shows the ego of an autistic child separated from the external environment by a sort of glass cage that can only be crossed by the sound that will open the first communication channel.

Fig. 3.2. shows the first step which is the search for the sound that penetrates through the glass wall and touches the autistic child's ego. This means that we have found a part of the child's ISO

**Therapeutic dynamics**

The starting point of the music therapy intervention is the child. The music therapist's task is to find ways to reach him, to penetrate the child's soul, but with discretion. The autistic child lives like under a bell jar, tries to make himself invisible, protects himself; transposes, but immediately withdraws into its shell. It is observed, in fact, that he perceives and takes note also very sensitively and in detail of reality even if immediately afterward he closes every contact in order not to have to perhaps react and behaves as if he had not seen, heard, understood nothing.

It is in this that he is hidden and closed that the music therapist tries to penetrate but with caution because attempting it with a wrong means would accentuate the child's resistance. In fact, while autistic in general, having the same characteristic behavior, they do not all behave in the same way for the same reason; therefore there is no common key and it is necessary to apply the individualized treatment.

At the beginning of the treatment the music can do very little; because the autistic child often rejects those sounds that are foreign to him and do not stimulate him.

The tactile movements that stimulate the senses are also foreign to him; its typical stereotype movement of beating anything with the back of the hand is a defensive movement, a movement of rejection contrary to the normal movement of the beating with the palm of the hand that foreshadows contact and includes exploring and taking.

The music therapist traditionally avoids using the voice in the spoken sense and tries to establish the first consensuality with the child trying to show him how, from his movements, from the stereotypes, from the mimicry, from the sounds emitted one can draw cues containing rhythms or melodic elements to build a possibility of the communicative score. The music therapist does not refer back to the child or the mirror but tries to interpret his bizarre score and read it musically, paying attention to all those out of tune or disharmony elements. In the case of a child whose activity continues to emit guttural sounds, the music therapist will try to evaluate the rhythm and melody of these sounds to see the variability of the expressive patterns present.

The order of the sequences will give indications about the difficulty of emitting the voice, in fact, the volume, the timbre, the false notes, the assonances will be evaluated to see if they constitute a primitive and original musical language, that is the degree of development of the autistic child. The music therapist, then, will be able to use these elements to structure playful proposals using mimicry, voice, movement and instruments in various ways. In fact, from the first meeting it is possible to observe links between the child's musical attitude and his pathology, links that lead the music therapist to a wider understanding of the problem of each child and the planning of therapeutic goals.

The music therapist will establish a goal from time to time since there is no predetermined goal. He will walk along with the child along the way, even on winding and steep roads, stopping where it would be appropriate to stop for a while. The music therapist will be able to make use of a therapeutic relationship at a musically receptive level in which the child will listen and focus attention on the sound or on a musically active level where the therapist will solicit and support dynamic involvement.

The common experience shows that many autistic children have a high level of attention towards stimuli of an acoustic or sound nature, therefore, by listening to certain rhythmic or melodic sequences one can often favor or establish some relationship with these children.

With regard to the use of musical instruments, it is generally observed, at least in the initial approaches, that the autistic child tends to develop a contact by provoking attraction, more than anything else, due to their geometric shapes, especially at a tactile level or sometimes even appropriating them through an oral report. The first task of the music therapist will, therefore, be to present and promote the knowledge of the tools available without any force.

Initially the musical expressions will serve to give the start to a tonic-affective exchange that will lead to the mutual completion of the sound identities, ISO, of the music therapist and of the child. Subsequently, mediated by music, the bodies of both will enter into synchronic vibration with sharing of perceptions and experiences able to arouse pleasant or annoying emotions or to evoke beautiful or unpleasant memories.

The child will thus begin to express himself freely through the body, the voice, the instruments and the music therapist will, in turn, be able to use the same expressive channels to build the relationship.

## The intervention project

Today we are establishing a mode of music therapy that is organized taking into account the complexity and variability of autism spectrum disorders, therefore we need to consider the peculiarities of the symptomatic framework of the child that can be traced to the following points:

- serious difficulties in activating communication, "the autistic lives in an unbreakable glass cage", both on the perceptive side and on the production side where there are cases of mutism or serious language disorders such as inarticulate sounds, stereotypes;

- implementation of other communication strategies through aggressive and traumatic behaviors due to atavism modalities such as kicking, rolling on the ground, biting, scratching, screaming, abandoning oneself to sudden excesses of anger anxious need to live in a stable and protective environment.

An important communication deficit emerges from the symptom picture, so the importance of interventions with non-verbal techniques is evident, first of all with music.

It is important to keep in mind that the difficulty or inability of these children to understand the codes that regulate any type of communication, causes a perception of the external world, as well as extraneous, very intense and invasive.

The closure in one's own inner world could be read as a necessity to defend oneself against excessive and unknown external stimuli. It is therefore essential to create a reassuring and welcoming environment, take a non-invasive attitude, apply non-verbal communication techniques, such as gestures, sounds with the voice or with musical instruments and mimic actions. This will make it possible to build a bridge of communication both with children without interest and apathy and with children who, instead, react intensely and in a disarray way to the sound stimuli.

In both cases, structuring the environment and activities according to rigidity criteria is certainly desirable to promote predictability, continuity, regularity, and order; on the other hand, an over-interventionist attitude of the music therapist could have disastrous effects.

A music therapy intervention could move in two ways:

- **communicative mode:** music intervenes on repetitive and stereotyped behaviors in a gradual way with the aim of establishing a communicative process,

- **affective mode:** the music in its melodic, rhythmic and timbric parameters acquires an affective value recognized and appreciated by the child.

The objectives of the music therapy project are therapeutic, therefore linked to the aspects of communication and relationship and rehabilitation type to enhance cognitive skills, attention and sensory-motor coordination. The project will also take care of increasing attention times and favor individual creativity that is so compromised in autistic children.

The final objective of the treatment will be changed, that is the possibility to modify or re-organize different areas of psychophysical functioning; "Change is the ultimate goal of all therapeutic intervention". The change takes shape and takes shape in terms of the intervention with respect to the specific individual characteristics of the departure of each subject.

In the music therapy intervention it is possible to identify various work phases linked to the different attitudes that the music therapist will take during the session.

## Technical elements

Indispensable, in order to proceed with an effective process of intervention in music therapy, is "to know clearly its two fundamental technical elements: the ideal music therapy laboratory and the instruments, of which, perhaps, it is not easy to dispose of in its entirety. It is possible, of course, to adapt it to institutional possibilities and according to specific clinical applications ".

## The music therapy laboratory

The music therapy laboratory is the physical space in which the sessions take place; it must be isolated acoustically because "in the non-verbal context, any external sound emission represents a disturbance capable of disturbing non-verbal communication".

We must preserve the same decoration throughout the experience so that the only thing that can change is the sound stimulus.

It is also necessary that the venue also offers a space for movement since body expression represents an activity closely connected to the therapy in which the subject is called to transfer music, sound and sound vibrations to his body. Benenzon underlines the importance of being able to use a wooden floor, in order to favor the transmission of sound vibrations.

Music, in the field of bodily expression, is translated into gesture, introducing more or less spontaneously a movement similar to dance, with liberating meaning.

The music therapy room is good enough to be large enough and collected enough to avoid the dispersion of attention. A size between forty and fifty square meters proves to be suitable; the excessive size could, in fact, be inadequate for the correct diffusion of the sound, creating problems of echoes or excessive reverberations with loss of intelligibility of the sound language. Furthermore, the room should be free of protrusions and dangerous edges.

The lighting of the room is planned so that it can be generalized or centered in a specific point; the use of diffused light and protected from the possibility of throwing objects is recommended. It is also expected that the room can be darkened to create games of brightness with specific materials or make games with shadows.

Benenzon provides a small table inside the music therapy laboratory with a metal container on top with a little water and a chair adapted to the child's stature. The container is made of metal so that if the child beats with his fingers it can produce sounds and vibrations; it is circular because it can make it turn.

There must also be a jug of water to be able to use it during experiments.

The use of water as an intermediary object is due to the following reasons:

- offers the child the possibility of non-verbal and non-oral response through play with water;

- it is a common element that the child lives daily, which has very pleasant regressive characteristics;

- it allows the music therapist to use movement and play techniques and allows contact with the skin by stroking with wet hands since these children accept this type of contact with fewer reservations.

In setting up the musical game we need rules, understandings, preliminaries, but also elements that are not calculated, outside the norm. It is in this very lively atmosphere that the activity takes place and the rules are represented by the field of action, the well-defined and not very confusing space, and in many cases also by the delimited time. The time allowed is approximately one hour a week since the weekly frequency can be considered quite favorable.

## The instruments

The means used in music therapy allow and suggest a multisensory intervention. It is commendable to transmit impulses in a penetrating, stimulating and fascinating way.

The means are not represented solely by instruments, they are also in ourselves, within us and around us. The necessary and used means are the musical instruments, such as the structured ones belonging to the Orff instrumentation and the self-built ones with different materials that lend themselves to different uses and to various transformations.

In some cases the material becomes the mediator of the relationship when a direct body contact could be premature and arouse rejection reactions. The environment should be well-stocked with sound and musical instruments, percussion instruments, wind instruments, string instruments, idiophonic instruments and other objects of various shapes, colors, and materials.

However, the instruments must be easily manipulated, easy to move and possess a peculiar sound power. Benenzon, among the necessary equipment in the music therapy laboratory, also includes a good stereophonic system, able to record sounds and offer multiple varieties of stimuli, so that it is possible to listen to and recognize significant moments for the individual child and that reinforce group identity.

As regards the instruments, then, Benenzon says that "every element capable of producing an audible sound or producing a movement capable of being experienced as a message, as a means of communication, will be an integral part of the music therapy tools".

## Structuring of the sessions

The success of a music therapy session depends primarily on the elasticity of the music therapist; he must hold the wires firmly in his hand, or possibly know how to loosen them at the right time so that the session can be profitable.

In the music therapy session the music therapist has available as work material the sounds, the silences, his own body, the noises, the music and the single elements that make up the music:

- the rhythm that acts on the intuitive sphere;

- the melody that acts on the sentimental sphere;

- the harmony that acts on the intellectual sphere.

The first session turns out to be the most important and decisive one here, in fact, the foundations are laid and a lot is already decided. The music therapist begins to learn about the child's ISO, on which he will gradually tune in. The first session can make the autistic child take a big step towards another perspective, bringing it to a change of relationships towards himself and others.

The true protagonist of the sessions is the child for whom the work of the music therapist can pass through the conduction, the mirroring, the going to the step, the stimulation, but in the end, the child will be the true actor-producer. Sometimes, even the silence of the music therapist can represent a precious therapeutic tool that can operate in order to restore integrity and visibility to the uniqueness of each child.

The dimension of silence, when it is not rejected in favor of an alleged and gratifying therapeutic action, represents a possibility of redefining the meanings attributed to one's own gestures and those of the child.

The following points are valid for the first session:

- **establishing trust:** we must, first of all, create a basis of trust to which the child's expectation contributes. The relationship of trust between music therapist and child will be realized in a contact, in a non-verbal agreement;

- **observe the child:** in order to examine what is in the child his visual, acoustic and social reaction will be observed. The secret to a good observation is to make room for the child so that it can accommodate its expressive freedom. This will be diagnostically very profitable;

- **structuring a therapy plan:** starting from the observations on the child the music therapist will proceed to the design of individual therapy plans with optimal therapeutic goals;

- **establishing a positive disposition in the child:** the charm of the action and the spirit that animates the musical game should lead the child to a state of enthusiasm.

The plan of the next session will refer to the previous one, the notes written by the music therapist after the first session will mark the essential moments. The subsequent sessions, in fact, will be organized according to the individual response of the children.

The moment of the reception takes a few minutes. The beginning of the activity has a path that leads gradually towards a crescendo of attention, up to the communicative intensity that characterizes the music therapy meetings. Each meeting will feature a welcome song and a song or final greeting dance.

Dance, where simple steps are used and you hold hands, can be a useful socializing means to overcome the fear of physical contact.

It will be proposed to listen to music, use instruments in a spontaneous or guided way, singing, physical activity, simple rhythmic or instrumental games, attention to different sounds or noises. The deliveries given on the use of musical instruments are verbal and non-verbal and have, depending on the moment, a connotation of directivity, semi-directivity, and non-directivity. Giving the child the possibility of using musical instruments is of great importance in music therapy; although it may happen that the child focuses his attention on non-functional elements such as the smell, the sensation that they give to the touch, the shape.

The interest shown by the child, however, expresses the awareness of the delimitation of boundaries and the distinction between self and other from itself. Furthermore, the fact that the child is able to make contact with an instrument often leads him to establish a first cause-effect relationship, a connection that autistic people usually do not grasp or grasp with difficulty, between the gesture aimed at the realization of sound and the sound from this resulting. It is necessary to create a context of sounds in which the child feels at ease and confident enough to express himself, to experience a wider range of emotions and to discover what is likely to be in a two-way communication relationship.

# The case of Giovanni: the first words after 15 years

After three and a half years of waiting, the first words. A long silence of Giovanni, an autistic boy of fifteen, from whom he came out thanks to his love for music.

A love that begins in his first years of life and that has introduced him to a new means of communicating, music therapy: a discipline that uses all the potential of the sound element within a therapeutic process.

"At three and a half years my son still didn't speak. He did not react to any external stimulus, closed in his silent world. One day I saw his gaze change, captured by something he was listening to there was the radio turned on and the notes of a song in the background that filled the room ".

Thus begins the story of Valeria, the mother of Giovanni, who, with music therapy, says, owes the joy of having heard her son call her mother.

A long journey that began in 1998 with the social co-operative "Le manielles".

*"From an early age, Giovanni has always been fascinated by everything that had a rhythm - says Valeria - I remember well how the expression on his face changed when he listened to music, his eyes were more attentive, he moved as if he wanted to dance and it seemed to me that he was trying to sing, but failed. So I inquired about the possibility of using music to help ailments like autism and I discovered, here in Parma, the association "The talking hands" in which my son started music therapy ".*

A child of only three years, Giovanni, able to choose his own care to break down that wall of silence that separated him from the whole world. A journey that continues today at the "Aias" center, now that that child has grown and is fifteen. "Since its first session it has been a success - continues Valeria -.

Every time my son finishes his music therapy time I see his face serene, relaxed. And this, for me as a mother, is the most important thing. After three months of attending music therapy sessions, Giovanni said his first words: mom and dad. And after six months he sang his first song: "I miss pee daddy."

Today Giovanni, thanks also to the help of other therapies, manages to communicate easily ".That of Valeria is sweet and longed for a story, which with satisfaction and meticulous details typical of each mother, tells the progress made by her son in these twelve years of music therapy.

# CONCLUSIONS

Music therapy is now applied in numerous clinical contexts and is also the subject of a growing interest even on the part of scientific circles that are more attentive to the verification of processes and outcomes.

To date, the music therapy intervention does not claim to reach conclusions that are rigorously and scientifically based in terms of method and fully valid in their statistical significance. Nevertheless, it can be stated that, in subjects suffering from the autistic syndrome, significant improvements were observed with the use of music therapy treatments since, it was found that a common characteristic, present in these subjects, is precisely the propensity towards music.

The music therapy intervention is aimed at improving the well-being and quality of life of autistic children and their families by acquiring alternative or augmented tools for verbal communication.It is not only music that is used in this type of treatment, but sound understood in its widest sense of movement-rhythm-sound.

The music must, therefore, be understood as a sound-human complex and its use is directed towards harmonization of the subject's personality. In autistic children music therapy has brought significant benefits both at a relational and cognitive level; in fact, music is a powerful and effective means of expression, capable of opening doors to the inner world of each child and helping him to get in touch with the outside world.

Music therapy allows us to observe, to listen, to perceive and to act by activating interpersonal communication. Precisely that communication that is so difficult and often unknown to autism carriers.

"Music is intelligible and untranslatable. And it is precisely because of this irreducibility that it can be the speech that manages to say something where language meets a limit ".

It should be borne in mind, however, that sound and music are not in themselves therapeutic, but must be used consciously and adapted to the individual child and to the peculiarity of his symptom picture.

In music therapy, sound and music delineate and structure that expressive and communicative activity which, interacting with ourselves and with each other, allows us to find and discover our most sensitive and profound nature.

For this reason, a good music therapist must not limit himself to the acquisition of theories, techniques, and methods, but must keep in mind that an important part of the path concerns the inner transformation of the person himself. The change must, first of all, involve the identity of the music therapist who needs it, before exploring and discovering himself and then readjusting and favoring the relationship with the child.

Today music therapy, thanks to the studies that have allowed its development, and thanks to its versatility, can be applied in various contexts such as in schools, hospitals, social centers, assistance centers, and communities.

It can be said that music therapy, despite being a relatively young and evolving discipline within the scientific landscape, can provide children with autism with a wealth of new skills and knowledge to facilitate them in addressing the complex issues posed by pathology, always according to the theories that the scientific community has approved, accepted and disseminated within the therapeutic proposals currently available.

Printed in the USA
CPSIA information can be obtained
at www.ICGtesting.com
LVHW021425010224
770630LV00002B/331